AF772845

FACING ME

Breaking the Bonds of Seizure Confinement

A Journey in Faith and Restoration

by Stephanie S. Sawyer

PublishAmerica
Baltimore

©Copyright 2002 by Stephanie S. Sawyer.

All rights reserved. No part of this book may be reproduced in any form without written permission from the publishers, except by a reviewer who may quote brief passages in a review to be printed in a newspaper or magazine.

First printing

ISBN: 1-59129-529-7
PUBLISHED BY PUBLISHAMERICA BOOK PUBLISHERS
www.publishamerica.com
Baltimore

Printed in the United States of America

This book is dedicated to

L. James Willmore, M. D.
Through whom I first experienced hope as he unlocked my bolted box;

to

Betty J. Shaw
For her compassion and gentleness in pulling me out of the box;

to

Eric, my husband,
For the security and companionship he has steadfastly offered like a beacon of light;

And beyond all
to

My Lord Jesus Christ
For putting these three in my path and constantly giving me His guiding Voice.

Table of Contents

Hope
is ours

if we will take it

and believe

Part I

A Set Way of Life

1. ADVENT OF A LIFESTYLE

There was never the remotest possibility in my mind that I could ever understand, much less attain, a lifestyle free from the bondage of regular seizure invasion. There was no other life for me. Frankly, I did not realize that I was consumed in an ill mindset which gripped my general view of myself. There had never been for me any other way of focus or understanding. The grip of chronic seizure intrusion was far more consuming than the seizures themselves. This entrapment which crossed every threshold of my activities in its surety of occurrence had me tightly locked in a vast realm of doubt and disbelief.

The only thing that I remember about those first series of seizures at age eleven is the accusations of being a bad child. I had been falling asleep in class. And thus the shame began. Days, maybe weeks, of these "falling asleep in class" accusations from my teacher penetrated my innocence. My reaction was confusion and a total loss of memory as to experiencing these episodes in the first place. Why was everyone on my case? I vaguely knew something was happening beyond my control. But I could only stupidly state, "I don't know" to the command of questions from my parents to this bizarre behavior from their normally highly obedient daughter. Finally, a trip to the doctor became their only course of action for answers to the puzzle.

Early on, these "spells" or episodes became known as black-outs to me. I would hear, "She keeps blacking-out." Or I would state, "I had another black-out." It is in these years of my early adolescence that my memory would begin to fail me, leaving huge gaps in my perception of events. Thus the mindset of inability set in.

I have no recollection of early doctors or EEGs

(electro-encephalographs testing). What I do remember is being told over and over that I would probably outgrow these black-outs. "Children usually do," stated the doctors. My EEG's were always normal. However, it was now declared that I was epileptic due to the regular pattern of my black-outs, which were now weekly, and I was placed on anticonvulsants immediately.

Where did this come from? It seemed to appear out of the blue. When questioned extensively my mother remembered a horrifying neonatal incident where my fever had pitched me into convulsion and loss of oxygen. Rushed into an oxygen tent for recovery I was given a spinal tap and various tests. Nothing showed up nor shed any light as to why I was convulsing. Now I know this is when the damage to my brain first occurred. But it lay dormant many years until adolescence struck.

My first bout with the anticonvulsant Dilantin was miserable: my gums swelled up painfully over my braces. Painful swelling persevered throughout weeks of misery. I was finally withdrawn off Dilantin and switched to Mysoline and Phenobarbital. Still, the black-outs continued. For years to come over various anticonvulsant combinations the seizures refused to subside becoming instead, my lifestyle.

Memories of my early adolescence are nearly non-existent. Even the most prominent figures in my life at that time outside of my family are empty slates on my mind. I know that I continued the piano training which I had begun at age nine. I had been declared "talented" very early, and my parents were advised to find the highest teachers possible for my training. Eventually, music and the piano would become my career. I was deeply enveloped in my love for music and piano, and yet, my memory will not bring up teachers of those early epileptic years. Big blanks form in my life which I believe are a result of a combination of the anticonvulsants as well as the interior brain damage causing the seizures.

The black-outs continued at no particular improvement.

They were never spoken of in my house despite their regular attendance. The shame of these disrupting, embarrassing episodes was like a ghost that was stuffed and locked in the closet never to be spoken of candidly or acceptingly. Therefore, I never knew what the black-outs were like since no one would talk to me about them. It was not until many years later when I met my future husband that I learned what these black-outs were really like. I only knew that I was having them about once a week.

From years of gathering data, I now know that the seizures were complex partial, "petit mal" we called them. I was always unconscious and they usually lasted a minute or two. I now know that they were staring spells with finger fidgeting and rocking, typical complex partial symptoms. I was always completely exhausted afterward. My inability to remember the simplest detail, my name, was humiliating, but common. Going immediately to bed was my only course of action, no matter what my prior activity had been, no matter its importance. Sleep was the only factor that could return me to my senses. Usually, I was shuffled away to my bedroom if I were at home. I have no recollection of how they were dealt with at school. Since they were quiet episodes, it would have been entirely possible to stay in place and remain inactive. Going "to sleep" in class was how they were diagnosed as I lay my head down on my desk following the black-out.

Shame enveloped me. Here was this obstacle of magnitude which never preannounced itself. It could happen anywhere, anytime. Due to the unspoken nature of this ghost in the closet at home, I learned to treat the black-outs in like manner though dreading the reality of their everyday occurrence which I knew could pop-out anywhere. Certainly, I understood rejection at home. This fear of rejection was now cast on my friends, for I knew, surely, someday, I would black-out in front of them. The inward sense of shame and inability grew and engulfed me with a dread of being found out, of having my secret forced out into the open.

Of particular disgrace was the tremendous self-proclamation and announcement of maturity that arrives with a driver's license at age sixteen. Not for me. Managing to hold my head up and equate myself as competent as my teen friends was a task I never accomplished. Though I had my regular teen cliques, I always knew from that ever-heated back burner of possible invasion that I was not good enough. I couldn't measure up. This was my life.

2. DEGRADING REALITIES

The impact of not driving was a serious degradation, a mark of serious flaw which I bore most personally. I internalized this inability so that it crossed over into my general outlook of capabilities in life. But the full scope of shame for not being a regular member of today's society in which we all care for our own needs did not truly hit me until I embarked onto independent living.

The social stigma of blacking-out on a date or among friends covered me with a low-grade sense of shame which permeated all of my activities. "What if…" seemed to be ever present even if buried in the recesses of my subconscious. Every week it would happen. At any time, any place. My aura of warning, a mere second of lapse in my mind, was not big enough nor dependable enough for me to take cover by removing myself to isolation. Within ten to fifteen seconds, the black-out was upon me and loss of consciousness hit me squarely over my whole being. My next cognizance would be minutes later in a dazed, confused, "Where am I? Who am I with?" In this state, which lasted a good number of minutes, I was unable to recall even my own name.

Though friends and boyfriends were always on a mission to assure me that I was acceptable, and even beautiful in my very being as a person, I was nevertheless filled with disbelief. The black-outs were continually locked in the closet of "pretend it's not there" in my original home, a closed subject for discussion unless an invasion hit among family members. Then, off to bed I was taken like a discard for not being good enough. Sympathy and understanding were not within my reach. And, most certainly, the word "seizure" was never used. What I did learn despite a few of these episodes was that I was not acceptable when these episodes struck; I had to be removed promptly and isolated until I returned to sanity.

My condition did not change for years to come. Early on, I had been filled with a vague hope that I would "outgrow" these black-outs. Any attempt of dialogue with my mother was answered with; "You'll outgrow them." Doctor's visits were serious enough that my father often attended and I knew something was royally amiss to claim his presence in the middle of a workday. Yet, I was still in the dark. EEG's kept painting "normal" graphs, my medicine never improved the regularity of the black-outs, and my parents kept meeting behind closed doors with my doctors as if I was a non-entity in the topic of discussion. Questions on the way home were usually met with, "We don't know anything," and the ray of hope in outgrowing them diminished quickly in spite of promises that I just had to wait.

My two younger sisters never spoke of these episodes to me. The whole house was so hush-hush. But I sensed talk behind my back, whether real or imagined, from those members of the family who had to open the closet door of "pretend it's not there" when witnessing a black-out. But I was kept outside of all dialogue, whether directly with my family or indirectly with my doctors. My sense of shame grew though I tried with all my might to be as normal as everyone else around me. Despite my efforts, still I disbelieved.

3. STEPPING OUT

I was happy to return to Texas where my roots were when I received admission to the college of my choice, Sam Houston State University, seventy miles north of Houston. The school was noted for music, and I had known for years that I wanted to expand my love and talents in music. It was also close enough to Houston and relatives that I could still keep a sense of home even though real home and parents were half way across the nation in Connecticut. I was fortunate to know solidly from the beginning with my piano skills where I wanted my life to head.

Though I knew I wanted to be incorporated in music, I never really thought I would have a high potent career as a performer or even a highly respected and developed instructor. Private instructors seemed to me to be a cut of the highest class with the highest refinement and expertise. This I would never have for I was already proven to be inadequate in my general view of myself. I couldn't measure up to general society much less be of the highest musical refinement. My talent was intact and I was going to expand it, and probably just teach on the side. But most of all I wanted the All American Dream. Surely, I'd find Mr. Dream Come True while I was in the process of securing a degree. And if my dream didn't formulate, I'd have my degree to fall back on to support myself. As so many freshman women dream of, I wanted my M-R-S. Then, I could enter into the womanly role of mother, cook, housekeeper, just as my own mother had done. I'd probably have a few students on the side.

I was broadly awakened to the complex and intricate world of music as I delved further and further into my field. Semester juries of piano solo performance in front of the piano faculty were my dread at the end of each semester. I was no performer and shied immediately away at the thought of anyone listening to me. I dreaded being heard in the practice rooms and was unable to entertain the aspect of sharing music. My music was strictly my own and I adored it, immersed myself in it, often as an outlet for my feelings of pain and inadequacy, of a haunting fear that I was an outsider.

But it was at this time of my life that I would discover a life changing reality, which later, in years to come, would draw me back into expression of my precious gift. My heart and vision were enlightened dramatically on one beautiful Saturday when I asked Jesus Christ to enter my heart as Savior and Lord. At this moment in time, Jesus became very real to me, a precious part of my everyday living, no longer an untouchable God. His Presence suddenly was touchable and my complete outlook on life shifted toward wanting to glorify God in my lifestyle. This enlightenment was a far cry from the judgmental god I was raised to believe in, a god who was only to be feared. The God who was only unapproachable suddenly became a reality in my life of love and joy as I saw His Light in a very personal way. This revelation would carry me through my darkest days ahead and later, bring me back to His very purpose for me.

The next years were joyous years for me, filled with the saturation of knowing the blessing of Christ's love and the blessing of His Spirit. I immersed myself in study of the Scriptures and solidly built friendships based on these lines. For the first time, it didn't seem to matter to my friends that seizures was a function of my life. I was truly happy, and yet, I knew in the deep recesses of my mind as I was in school that there was a monumental obstacle in front of me.

Despite my grand awakening as a child of God, my sense of self and beauty therein were still seriously depleted. I continued my music studies moving eventually to the University of Houston. But I dreaded that final year of school that was becoming closer and closer. It held an obstacle I could not touch for it was certain to defeat me. As a music major I was forced into this peril or I could not graduate. I had to give a recital. My black-outs were still a weekly visitation as they had been for years. So far, they were no terrible disruption to the general public, for my lapses were not convulsive nor did they draw attention when they occurred. They continued to be quiet, minimal body involvement, carrying on for several minutes after which my memory would be blown away. They were somewhat easy to hide on a college campus where students are diverse and self-focused. But I could never outguess when they might occur. Suppose it was the stage!

It didn't matter that the likelihood of a black-out on stage during a recital might be somewhat minimal. What mattered was that it could occur. I felt locked down in inability. Shame grasped me. I did not know how to throw off the shackles of disbelief. Outside of not being capable to obtain a driver's license this was the first event of reality in my life compounded by epilepsy that seriously cast me into a box of defeat. I was drastically limited by the presence of black-outs in my life and my humiliation on never-talk-about-it in my family carried over into my general outlook for my life. I could go nowhere. I could do nothing. And so I did nothing but retreat from college when I was face to face with that threshold of musically "coming-out," the awesome senior recital. My progress in life stopped dead, and I retreated, despite my conversion, to a more serious sense of shame and self-doubt than ever before. I was trapped, and there was no way out.

4. A SAFE PLACE

Eric was my first safe place. With him, it didn't matter if I openly had a seizure. He was my first assurance of full acceptance and even compassion. The word epilepsy didn't scare Eric. The word seizure didn't terrify Eric though it took years for me to break down the barriers of horror, the "pretend-it's-not-there background barriers," and use the word. But I was prevalent thanks to Eric's free acceptance and encouragement. Eric has always been my free shield of safety. To him, I was just as special as any fully healthy person, and I was not meant to be rejected for a flaw in the system. To him, I was special and he became the whole world to me. He became my first ray of light in a darkened self-image, and a beacon of hope to my shattered sense of self. He believed in me!

I talked to Eric about everything. We met at the University of Houston and I quickly lapped up his encouragement and calm, peaceful friendship like a thirsty sponge. I had never known anything like it. Eric was my safe place, a haven of belief. I couldn't shake him with any crisis or tale of defeat. He just wouldn't accept my bleakness of future, but instead, tried all the harder to convince me that I was beautiful and had tremendous gifts to be shared.

Eric liked to sit on the floor during my practice sessions, my daily ritual with the piano, and study. He was the only one I ever felt safe enough with to allow hearing all the drudgery of musical refinement. Yet, he enjoyed it. He seemed to bask in our togetherness. The mode of acceptance and his enjoyment pierced my heart with a comfort and friendship level far surpassing any I had ever known. I did not know I was falling in love with him.

Eric did not meet my preconceived criteria for Mr.

Prince Charming. His earthy kindness and somewhat rustic background did not fill the prescription for the suave, sophisticated, debonair leader that I had in mind. Foolish concept! I had the whole world at my fingers. Eric was everything I had ever truly wanted and more. I was already deeply in love with Eric, and I soon realized I needed to bury the foolishness of my preconception. Eric listened to me like no other. His kindness was like none I had ever touched. I perceived Eric as wise in his philosophies and admired him for such. Eric was what I had been looking for. His only detriment was in taking so very long to make up his mind and act on things. But I knew the wait would be worth it. Over a year into our courtship, he finally popped the question knowing full well my standing. We were married the next year.

5. ENTRAPMENT AT HOME AND WORK

I settled in quickly and happily to the role of homemaker. I continued my employment in banking which I had started the previous year. I had resigned my musical skills in defeat knowing I was unable to meet that final criteria, the recital. I had left school, my music degree incomplete, and found myself now without a piano. Suddenly, I had to make my way in the world. Numbers had a particular attraction for me, which is not surprising considering their correlation to music, so I began a career in accounting clerical work and bookkeeping in the year of Eric's and my courtship. Numbers worked well for me in my highly detailed and trained eye. I continued in bookkeeping and accounting after our marriage, but found myself swiftly leaving behind all that I loved, music and the art of expression.

Two children were born within the first four and a half years of our married life, Emily, my angel, and Aaron, my heartthrob. I was determined to raise them completely myself, so I left my work to give them my total devotion. I was ecstatic to be a mother, but found myself seriously confined with no driver's license. Trips to the pediatrician had to be arranged in favors by friends. All grocery trips had to await my husband's presence. Even emergency medical situations, and Emily had numerous, were at the mercy of me finding transportation through another. We lived tightly on a budget so I made the most out of the city bus system, but even this mode of transportation was highly limiting in time and destination. I eventually grew to feel more and more ashamed that I was unable to provide for my children in the simplest family pleasures. A trip to McDonald's was unthinkable. A sudden run to the grocery store was impossible. Social gatherings were based solely on the willingness of friends to cater to my limitations. I was completely of the mind that I was a burden to others around me in my constant need. In my children's toddler years, I worked out a plan with a friend to visit a grocery store together once a week on a certain day. But I never actually believed I wasn't limiting my unchained friend by my need for a ritualized agenda. And though her compassion may have been abundant for me, somehow my background of shame would not allow me to believe it. Surely, I was not really equal with all the other young families around me, for they could supply for their families and I could not.

As Emily and Aaron became involved in school, I saw the need to return to work. Eric and I had purchased a piano, and I adored playing it though somewhat limited in my repertoire with no formal lessons. I remembered that this could never be my life despite my love for music. I didn't really have what it takes. So, once again, I sought accounting work and was able to secure a job in a local bank. Over the next several years, I remained in banking working in various departments, never quite happy with my position at a desk all day long. My numerical skills were high which I, once again, attributed to my musical background, but I never seemed to blend in with the clerical office environment. I dragged on with a lack of satisfaction, merely doing my duty toward my family. A life of drudgery and social inability seemed to be swallowing me up.

Several years into my accounting career my position took a nose-dive into one of the most drastic positions of my life. The devastation of this period would become a turning ground for me though all I knew for months was absolute rejection and despair. I had hit rock bottom and there was no way out.

I had been enjoying a new position as assistant to the controller in a local real estate firm. My skills were high and appreciated as such. My Galleria office overlooking ritzy Post Oak Boulevard looked out over the city I loved in a panoramic view. I was happier than I had ever been in my career, and the office manager repeatedly let me know how very pleased the management was with me. I had surpassed their expectations in a very short while. My career finally seemed launched and I was inhaling the sweetness of success. Then the seizures hit.

There were several in a row over several days. It was uncommonly frequent though not unheard of that I should have a few within hours of each other. On at least two occasions, I had to retreat to the couch in my office to rest out the disorientation in the aftermath. Management bolted. My forewarnings of rare occurrence with recuperation in the form of a coffee break, my usual stance and solution at the past bank position, became unbelievable, and I was instantly relieved of duty. As I protested in disbelief, the manager quoted that the company could not be held liable if I should fall due to a seizure. It did not matter how high my skills had been. It did not matter that I never fell from having seizures. The former praise given me did not seem to matter. What mattered was that I was epileptic though I had forewarned them so. Fear reigned. I was fired point blank.

No other employer had ever treated me this way. I had numerous years in banking, at least three years with one bank. As always, the seizures popped up weekly, but were not that noticeable since they were more like staring spells and finger fidgeting. I had never run into any difficulty before because I was so frank with my employers. But it is true there was a fluke that week that caused a set of seizures. I was instantly rejected.

The stigma of being faulty, not good enough, threw me into an emotional collapse far surpassing my power to deal with. I had once received high praises from this very company that instantly fired me for seizures on the job. There was no ADA in that year, 1990 or so. But, even so, my faith kept me from considering a lawsuit, which would have been very difficult to prove.

Instead, my career came to a screeching halt and sent

me into tumbling depression. I could barely function at home much less initiate a job search. I could not move for the darkness this disorder, epilepsy, was casting on my life. I could have no hope of winning. I could not conceive of success. I was doomed to shame and inability by the very presence of these uncontrollable seizures. It was no use trying. I was ensnared. I could not see then that my career devastation would be only the beginning of a journey of hope and light far surpassing anything I could imagine. This, too, would be redeemed.

Part II

A Doctor Who Believes

6. BEGINNING FOOTSTEPS

It took a tragedy and personal devastation for me to encounter and eventually embrace the man who would change my life forever. It took complete despair from my crashed career for me to surrender my future, my brain, my ultimate functioning ability to another human. The trust I grew to have in this one doctor alone had to be monumental for me to surrender to such a radical notion, brain surgery.

In my initial devastation over my crashed career I reached out for the first time to the Epilepsy Foundation's local chapter in Houston. Never before had I felt so marked with a handicap as to believe I had a reason to be associated with them. My old schooling of "pretend-it's-not-there" stated, "It's not so bad that you should need *them*!" But now I was humbled to the core, marked as inadequate, rejected for something beyond my control. I was suddenly the subject of discrimination.

The Foundation was quick to come to my aid with comfort, understanding, information, and more friendship than I can ever repay. I am ever indebted to Donna Stahlhut, Director at our local chapter in Houston, for the information and companionship forwarded. Suddenly, my isolation was broken, and I was truly among friends, among people who honestly understood the reality of seizure invasion and spoke of it commonly, out of the closet.

It was at that first encounter at the Foundation that I was given a blessing that would change the course of my life. Pam Jones, a staff member of the Foundation and personal friend, gave me the name of Dr. L. James Willmore, a research expert on new anticonvulsants.

"He is the founder and director of the Texas Comprehensive Epilepsy Program," she explained. "Associated with the Texas Medical School," she went on, "Dr. Willmore is constantly researching new drugs, and is the ultimate resource on seizure control. His expertise is unmatched. Besides," she continued, "he's just starting research on a new drug and is looking for study candidates. Perhaps you could be a part of his program."

When I resisted in my despair due to lack of insurance coverage and my inability to cover charges, she continued to extend hope. "There are no charges for study patients. Go see Dr. Willmore."

And with that, the beginning footsteps toward a major miracle began.

7. WAIT AND SEE

Dr. Willmore never seemed to tire of saying it, "Wait and see!" My first visit was filled with his mirth and a medical hope such as I had never encountered. I had long grown used to passive surrender to mediocre control of my seizures by my previous doctors. "Accept it," they shrugged off. "You're in pretty good shape for being epileptic. Your ability to function is pretty normal." These were actual words I heard from former doctors; not, "Let's lick this thing!" But Dr. Willmore: His zest and mirth were unlike any doctor's characteristics I had ever encountered. Who was this man that he was so spirited? Who was he that he could possibly do anything for me?

Yes, Dr. Willmore was beginning a new study on the research drug Felbamate. Yes, I seemed to be a good prospect, uncontrollable seizures. But, first, I would have to succumb to an aggressive clinical testing of established anticonvulsants despite my previous drug history and their lack of control. Documentation of every seizure and medication was of absolute necessity. We would start with Dilantin. No matter the adverse side affects suffered as a child, we must follow the program. The study required that every suitable anticonvulsant be tried. Dr. Willmore assured me that he expected no progress in control, but the study required it. Eventually, we would move to the study drug once we had established a medical history.

Then Dr. Willmore, in his aggressive academic style, moved one step further. The bottom line, he stated, was that he thought I would be a probable candidate for brain surgery. If during the Felbamate study, I received no progressive control, then we would look in-depth at the possibilities of corrective surgery for me.

I was stunned. Yet hope dared to burn. It was a far cry,

a radical move. Yet, this doctor had such mirth as he spoke of it. The pleasure in his face from having seen such positive results in post-surgical patients spread over my soul like a ray of hope, a beam of pure light. This man was suddenly saying, "There is a way." And his smile and countenance warmed my heart in the midst of the drasticness of his suggestion. "But wait and see," he continued. "We'll start you on the study right away."

8. A REMARKABLE PROGNOSIS

As forecast, I spent the next year or so in an aggressive search for seizure control through established anticonvulsants. Among these were Dilantin, Depakane, Depakote, Tegretol, and several others. All failed to make any difference in my weekly invasion of unconsciousness. However, Dr. Willmore continued his mirth and jolly output, knowing it was only a matter of time and documentation before he would walk me through a magnificent journey. I succumbed to just trying the drugs and keeping track of every damn seizure, an easy task for me with my detailed bookkeeping skills. Maybe the Felbamate would bring some improvement.

I was still unemployed through this phase, and the impact on my sense of inadequacy was great and cumbersome. Every prospective employer's decline reiterated that I didn't measure up, that I was a misfit, and I took this message to heart. I stumbled in and out of temporary assignments, forever fighting to meet our stretched monthly budget. The strain I felt was without relent and I believed myself to be a major burden to my family of four in my inability to hold and sustain a job.

At last, the time came to turn to the study drug, Felbamate. I should continue to document all seizures, call them in to Dr. Willmore's office, and look for any adverse side affects. Long a lover of detail, it was easy for me to document the seizures, their length and the events surrounding them. I never found any common thread for them or spark which ignited them, certainly not stress. Only my menstrual cycle seemed to have a claim on their presence, and that not always.

In the weeks ahead, I noticed a remarkable drop in the amount of seizures I was having. Once I boosted up to the full dose of Felbamate which was nearly toxic for me I noticed a strong departure from the weekly invasion. Suddenly, the lapse of time between them boosted to three weeks. Joy! I was receiving far better control! Never had I known such a dramatic increase of control! No medication had ever had such profound affect on me and I was overjoyed at this newly found victory.

But not Dr. Willmore. To be certain, he was pleased for me that my seizures were less frequent. He was also grateful that I was such a good study participant due to my accurate record keeping. “The best,” he continually bragged. He griped about participants who did not keep diligent records, and he praised me for my accuracy. But he did not stop there.

No, Dr. Willmore was not satisfied with finding good study results. He wanted more. The seizures were still a regular pattern of invasion in my life and he would not be still for having just achieved improvement. He was convinced that he could bring me a life of freedom, a life not invaded by seizures. He believed he could bring me health in a way I had never known it. He clearly was not satisfied to accept my joy over increased control with the Felbamate. All I could do was hang onto his shirttails and make the decision to wholly trust him. He wanted to fight my battle and he radiated confidence in winning. It was now my decision to let him do it, and surrender disbelief.

He began to talk to me about brain surgery. He talked so fast, so knowingly. Yet, never did he rush out of the room. He always stayed for as long as I wanted, and “then some,” answering everything I could possibly think of. Dr. Willmore took time with me of which I am so grateful.

He began to tell me that he thought I would be an excellent candidate for the procedure. Of course, it would require a lengthy and intense examination through in-patient hospital testing at the Texas Comprehensive Monitoring Unit in Hermann Hospital. This would determine the source and place of initiation of the seizures. Was I willing?

Suddenly it was happening so fast! How could this happen? I balked. I came in for a check-up. He started talking surgery. Now he wanted to check me in for in-hospital testing. Though I wanted to agree, I certainly had no way to pay for it. I was unemployed, had no savings, and felt destitute. "Not to worry," he proclaimed. I came to know in the months ahead that this was his favorite saying. "Not to worry," he constantly threw back at me when I voiced my concerns all be it physical, financial, or any other insurmountable hardship. He gloried in holding out beacons of light and hope to me where I had once only known defeat.

Dr. Willmore immediately assured me that I would be provided for. Provided for?! Me?! How could this be? At this point Dr. Willmore began to talk about the Texas Rehabilitation Commission. He would talk to Iliana deJuan, a Senior Counselor closely involved with his work. "Who is this?" I puzzled, not knowing a thing, some strange name, some strange agency. Why would they want to have anything to do with me? I was an unknown, a failure in the world at large. Why would anyone be interested in me? "Not to worry," I kept hearing. His belief was more than I could fathom. But I gave him my permission and went home too marveled to think straight. Somebody out there wanted to fight for me, wanted to talk some agency into supporting me. In my mind, I envisioned Dr. Willmore having to prepare an argument, prepare a case to this woman, this agency. Could it really happen? Was brain surgery really within my grasp? Could I possibly be set free? It was too much for me to consider. But I had learned to trust Dr. Willmore. His mirth and the twinkle in his eye mixed with my encounters with his expertise had become a strong foundation for me. If he said it, then I knew there was truth. Now there was only to establish "Could it be for me?" I gave up trying to understand it and could only hold onto the ray of hope Dr. Willmore afforded me. My wait had begun.

9. COULD IT BE?

Marvelous were the words that came to me of approval for admission into the Texas Comprehensive Epilepsy Program located in Hermann Hospital in the Texas Medical Center. Dr. Willmore had just proven to me his power, and from then on, I knew that I would be supremely taken care of. "Not to worry" was a touchable concept.

When I arrived at 4 Jones Pavilion for the week long testing where TCEP resides I was suddenly immersed in seizure victims all around me though they were not acting so. I marveled at the "no big deal" attitude I witnessed from the other patients when they spoke of their seizures. How could they feel this way? Each was in his own room, "all wired up," or some in the community room with family members at hand.

They were each there for twenty four-hour surveillance of EEG monitoring waiting for that blessed seizure to occur in order to locate its point of origin. Most all of them were raving about Dr. Willmore, how he was giving their lives hope again. This doctor was clearly devoted to overcoming obstacles and was using all his capacities to do so. Now it was my turn to enter the TCEP community.

10. NIGHTMARE ASSIGNMENT

"Have seizures," I was told by Dr. Willmore. "We want to locate what part of your brain they're starting from." If the seizures were initiating from one area, I would be a good surgical candidate; if they were widespread, I would not.

The EEG technician, Pam Zanek, wired me up and kindly explained the 24 hour monitoring. I was to summons the nurses whenever I knew or felt that a seizure was coming on. My medicine was reduced immediately, and I was basically to lie around and wait for "it" to happen.

It began to happen without much wait. This time I was on TV as they happened. Every grunt, every fidget, every symptom was getting filmed to be analyzed next to the EEG with it. Where did this seizure come from? I remember on one particular occasion when I was blown away with disorientation following a seizure that Dr. Willmore waltzed into the room gleefully whooping, "That was a great seizure!" I was so taken aback by his enthusiasm when I was left in the mire by it all. I was unable to process any information for hours afterwards and I felt dangerously disoriented. The scope of rattling in my thinking abilities was enough to really scare me, and I spoke about it that day with a dear friend while in a fog the whole while.

But the week finally closed and Dr. Willmore got his information. Yes, I was the perfect surgical candidate. Those complex partial seizures were "classic," as he put it. He pinpointed my right temporal lobe. Years later, he told me that he used the film of me having seizures in his classes with his students, my seizures were so classic. Our victory now was that my seizures were coming from one local spot, a reachable spot with the scalpel. There was one more test, but we definitely wanted to arrange for the surgery. Was I willing to move forward?

Willing – to be healed?

Willing – to have my brain cut into, my center of processing, the seat of my personality?

I swam in conflict.

I was horrified. What could happen to me? The worst jumped out. Suppose that I lose some of my functioning. Perhaps giving up the seizures would mean sacrificing part of my regular abilities.

My mind endlessly ran the "suppose" list, until I reminded myself how Dr. Willmore had come into my life. For I believed it was no coincidence that I was led to this man in my moment of despair.

As my "suppose" list ran on through my head, Dr. Willmore waiting patiently beside me to make up my mind, I thought how badly he wanted me to be completely healed, more than any other doctor I had ever known. My mind returned to his valiancy in belief, and his ability to bring to fruition that desire for improvement. Then, too, I felt I must believe. He was swaying me.

Questions arose.

Money... My ability to Think … Function… Process …

"Not to worry," "Not to worry," "Not to worry."

He spent a long time with me until I was satisfied.

And I finally believed. Not because he had twisted me into it, but because he had been gentle with my doubt, but firm in his conviction.

"That part of your brain is not functioning anyway," he explained. At first, he tossed out the idea of scraping the scarred tissue away. "We'll just have to go in and see what's there," he continued. Once again, I resigned to him knowing security with him much as a small child does with a father. Indeed, TCEP is a family, and L. James Willmore is the father of it all.

He instructed me to go home and wait for a phone call

from DeeDee who would receive my surgical date. Little did I know that phone call would be six months down the road! The wait and anticipation of surgeons going into my brain was one of the most anxious times of my life.

11. WAIT FOR THE LORD

BE STRONG, AND LET YOUR HEART TAKE COURAGE; YES, WAIT FOR THE LORD.

Ps. 27:14

The word 'wait' will forever be a changed concept to me. I believed the Lord had opened mighty doors for me to bring me to this place in my life where this spectacular event could burst forth. Now, I was needing every tool of spiritual strength I had ever learned in my Christian walk as this waiting period extended. My imagination in the meantime, never wanting for creativity, had to be quieted continually through peaceful music. I literally had to shut myself down from much social engaging and place myself in a completely serene environment to overcome my nervousness over that which I was about to undertake. Surgeons going into my brain! I didn't have Dr. Willmore to reassure me everyday, and I had no idea when DeeDee might call and tell me to come in.

The testing had been in January '92. Weeks and months turned into agonizing waiting. I leaned on Eric mightily during this time. I have not spoken much of Eric, but he was such a strength, such a gentle force of love and encouragement. I always knew I could fall back on Eric. He, too, was excited about my upcoming opportunity and encouraged me with Dr. Willmore, to believe that there was full healing available for me. Eric's understanding was sweet when I was testy and most difficult to be with.

Though I may have leaned on friends in many instances of crisis, this situation was one I could only swim the waters alone. I knew with all my heart that the Lord had opened mighty doors for me, and it was for me to continue to believe. Questions and wonderment put forth to me by friends only upset my natural guarded boundaries so I secluded myself as much as I could. I believe I removed myself from all other stressors because this one alone was so extreme that it demanded all my energy and resolve to handle. I wrote out the Scripture, "Wait for the Lord; Be strong, and let your heart take courage; Yes, Wait for the Lord," Ps. 27:14 and set it on my bedside where it would be a constant reminder of the source of all of my strength. I am thankful for the music of John Michael Talbot, a Franciscan monk, during this time. I knew that I had to throw myself completely in God's Hands, and that Dr. Willmore was His tool of service.

DeeDee finally did call, but it was not until late Spring. My surgical date now stood at June 15th. I was to be admitted a few days early for neuropsychological assessment and also for the WADA test which Dr. Willmore kept talking about. This final critical test would assess the functioning ability of each side of my brain, of the temporal lobes. It would tell how dependent I was on my right temporal lobe for functioning in any capacity before surgeons decided to yank it out from their EEG and MRI findings. By now, I also had a PET (Positron Emission Tomography) scan, and I reveled in the Polaroid-like picture of my brain the technician sent home with me. I could look at a picture of my brain in my own bedroom and note the activated part that was causing more trouble during the testing. Wow!

It was not until I reached my hospital room a few days before my scheduled surgery that Dr. Willmore had the gall to announce he just might be out of town a few days in the up-coming days. He wanted to warn me. Of course, he was not the surgeon, but I was horrified at the thought of my rock of Gibraltar not being around while surgeons were drilling holes into my skull and going into my brain. He teased me that he had really wanted to be around for "this one," and that if he didn't completely trust the team there'd be no way he'd leave. But he had the utmost trust for them and assured me I was really going to like my neurosurgeon, Dr. Guy Clifton. What could I do now but again decide to place my trust in this man, this doctor, who wanted so much to fight my battle for me, to see me win, and give me the health I had never had. All I had to do was yield.

12. FINAL CONFIRMATION

My full and complete peace of mind, my faith in the upcoming operation only two days ahead, was utterly achieved through the results of one test, the WADA. Thus, I was not so utterly dependent on my faith in one man, my doctor, James Willmore. Once I had experienced in my own brain the functioning abilities this test challenged, I knew, I KNEW, I was safe for this operation. I rested.

In layman's terms, while prepped extensively ahead of time, I was quizzed thoroughly by a team of doctors on memory. The doctors had visited me the previous day and given me a series of patterns, visual and aural to memorize. Being a visual person, I had asked them for the ability to take notes during the briefing. "No go," was the answer. So I depended on every source of memory skill I had developed over time, using mental games and repetition to drive into my mind the patterns put before me.

During the WADA, named for the doctor who invented the test, half of my brain was put to sleep and I was quizzed on my memory skill on my functioning side. This lasted a few minutes, roughly, six, and then the reverse side was deadened so that each side could be tested. When my damaged right side was deadened, I have been told, I was quite keen and answered all questions on memory far better than expected. I can remember to this day a fair part of that testing, and even some of the graphical displays used in the testing. My speech at the time was sluggish, but I was highly aware of that. When the left side was deadened and I was dependent on the scarred right temporal lobe, I started out keen but grew unresponsive to the point of no response for ten to fifteen minutes. I was told the doctors poked and prodded, thereby proving my complete reliability on my left temporal lobe for memory skill. It also proved how dysfunctional my right temporal lobe really was. Don't just scrape it. Take it out! I was now ready for the surgeon's drill. Monday was only two days away.

13. THROUGH THE TUNNEL

"It's all over, Babes!" cried my mother as she burst into the Neuro Intensive Care Unit at my first sign of post-operative consciousness and feebly cried out, "Mama." My husband has never comprehended that first declaration nor hardly forgiven me, and surely, he deserved better after nearly twelve years of marriage. But it was a sign of what was to come in the scramble my brain had just been thrown into. We, nor I, had not been forewarned of this. I only knew that the seizures would go away. Little did I realize what would happen to my immediate comprehensive skills once I left the hospital.

I was a rat in NICU: all those tubes, all that prodding, that stupid turban. Where was Willmore?

It seemed that every five minutes a nurse was coming in asking me who the President of the United States was. What day is it? What's your name? One came in and called me "Steph," and to my cognizance, I roared out at her like a lion in anger, so great is my detest for the shortened name. Eric corrected me weeks later saying I could hardly mutter. But my spirit was alive and kicking. Of course, I had no skill to think to control myself. I was purely reactive. But I still had my natural born fire inside, my passion, the passion Willmore loved, and I turned it against the nurses. I wanted out of NICU and I wanted out NOW! Give me my room back; get this turban off my head!

This, of course, is some exaggerated memory, but Dr. Clifton did remove me fairly pronto (Tuesday) to my private room. He reported a "super surgery" and stated his pleasure at my advance. The right temporal lobe was severely scarred once they actually got into my brain and saw the full scope of the early damage. He expected nothing but full recovery for me. As pleased as I was, I was craving Willmore. When does he get back into town?

I was nestled among Eric, family, and friends for the next week in horrible pain and headaches with jaw aches (from the cut jaw muscle just below the lobe) unlike any I had ever experienced. But the man didn't show up for another week, and then it was on particularly good timing.

The previous night while with friends, I suddenly found myself uncontrollably going into major convulsions. This was the first sign of any seizure occurrence. There were three convulsions, not seizures as I knew them, and I never lost consciousness, but watched horrified as my body tossed and writhed in uncontrollable jerks. I could not stop it nor cry out. I gasped on my own saliva, choking in need of air. Once they had stopped, I had to be sedated I was so panicked at the experience. Where was Willmore?

My friends, Rob and Martha, who had been visiting, were stalwarts of strength to me following those convulsions. Rob instantly took my hand and grabbed my gaze with authority during my panic. He would not let me go under with the horror of this terrifying behavior my body demanded. Twisting, jerking, choking, stiffening, I had not experienced this before. I was collapsing in fear and defeat from my prior triumph which we had just been candidly speaking about and rejoicing in. Then, suddenly, this disgrace was over me! But Rob, and now Martha, his wife, would not let me fall spiritually. They commanded me to remember whose I was, the Lord's Himself, and He would not abandon me.

A doctor was petitioned through the flooded streets of Houston. I was told he would have to canoe his way in. Then I was wheeled downstairs for an immediate CT scan to check for air bubbles and blood clots. Rob and Martha never left my side, and I truly needed their comfort, strength and reassurances when it seemed that my whole world had just come crashing down on me. I had just had the worst type of seizures I had ever encountered in my life. Indeed, they were major convulsions though I had been promised victory and health. Where was Willmore?

The CT scan came out clean, and I was told by the doctor on-call that there would be no more. My family had been summoned through the floods, and I only found true relief in Eric's arms. Eric gave me the assurance that the seizures were so different that he believed they were not a threat. This was a valuable insight and a precursor of the medical insight my doctor would give me. But still, I had to hear it from Willmore. Where was he?

Those convulsions happened on a Sunday night, six days following my operation. Dr. Willmore's voice finally resonated through the halls of TCEP on Monday morning as he started rounds. I jumped out of bed, though still learning to walk again, and dashed as best as I could to find him. There he was in another patient's room with his team.

He looked up with that ever-cute little grin on his face. He was glad to see me; he laughed. But he forced himself to back down saying he'd be down to my room in a few minutes. He didn't want to break the routine of room flow in his rounds. Darn it, Willmore! I retired to my room at ease that my security was back.

When he waltzed in quite a while later with his crew his announcement was, "You did like a champ!" He proclaimed last night's convulsions a 'fluke,' the MRI, which I had taken this morning, had proven that. And, therefore, he was sending me home. Today. "Today!" I balked. Then, he continued, "We'll have a party when you get your driver's license!" He kept impressing, "You're doing great!"

Then he gave me a visual picture which was so very helpful in many of my dark days which were to come. He said what I had been through is like the equivalent of being run over by a 16-wheeler. So he alerted me to crying jags, commanded me to "WALK!" and, as always, reminded me he was just a phone call away.

Part III

The Dark Night

PRELUDE

No one told me it would be like this.
No one forewarned me of the blackness I now know.

Everyone celebrated, myself included. And they are still celebrating. And they should.

But I am left alone. I had a rude awakening – an awakening too painful to recall without determination to do so. But I must. It is part of my story.

All I expected was a victory too big to grasp. And, indeed, that happened. But much more accompanied that victory. A depression deeper and larger than anything I have ever touched. A depression far outside the field of what I would allow in the view of my victory. How could I dare cry? How could I dare allow myself to be so overcome?

Ah! But I had no choice. It happened. The forces against me were so large – larger than any I could describe – or explain – larger than what I could handle.

So all became black. And I felt as if I was walking in a death.

This is not what was supposed to happen. This is not right. The epilepsy is gone. Doom and despair should not be my answer. What has happened to me? Will I ever see daylight again?

Daylight
I must wait for the sunrise.
I must think of a new life,
And I mustn't give in.
When the dawn comes
Tonight will be a memory, too,
And a new day will begin.

Trevor Nunn
After T. S. Eliot

14. IDENTITY CRISIS

The pain was intolerable at first; the commotion unreal. My children were frightened of their moaning mother and I was at a loss for comfort of any kind. Sleeplessness allowed me no respite when the house closed down at night other than lying around. I quickly went into overload over the simplest of chores, as if I was retarded and had to stop midstream or slow to a ridiculous pace. Reaching under the sink to pull out the dish soap and wash a dish was a major affair in that first week. My mind felt blasted by the details involved in just opening up the bottle of soap, then squirting some minor amount into the dish, pushing back down the top and replacing the soap under the sink. I was completely unable to explain all this to Eric. Words completely escaped me, and I lived in confusion. Thankfully, he sensed my difficulty and took care of me. My comprehensive skills took weeks and months to rebuild. I kept thinking of being hit by that 16-wheeler and realized this was what Dr. Willmore was warning me about.

Within a few weeks of my surgery, I walked into the bathroom one morning, looked myself in the mirror and realized I didn't know who I was. What was my identity? The scars over my right ear seen by the bald spot the size of my palm shouted out I was no longer epileptic. But that was yet to be proven. Looking in the mirror, I wondered who I was looking at. At least beforehand, I knew the ritual. Now, I didn't have a clue. So much of my identity had been wrapped up in this one aspect of me. I was still jobless – I was really of no importance to anyone other than my family, EXCEPT to Dr. Willmore. I was his #1 Felbamate study patient, and I know more than that. Now, he was walking right out of my life. Who was I?

My first quest was to establish myself in dependable employment. For months prior to my operation I had jumped around temping in clerical accounting work though the work was highly unsatisfactory. Added to this was the increasing financial strain my loss of steady employment had put us under. For the first time in our lives, Eric and I were actually being threatened by creditors. We had built a lifestyle based on two steady incomes which had been dependable for years. Then suddenly, with my release from Fuller Real Estate, I was no longer able to find employment and hardship became a reality.

Dr. Willmore had told me that I had been hit by that 16-wheeler. The functioning and processing my brain needed in recovery took weeks, not a few days. Emotionally, it took months for me to psychologically get back on my feet. The entire time, I was trying to sort out who I was, which way I wanted to go, and how to relate to myself in a new way. I had no help at first, only spinning thoughts, and a lot of demanding creditors on the telephone. In the midst of this was a jubilant wanting to exalt God, and gleefully crying out to everyone on every corner who would listen, "I've been healed! I've been healed! Touch my scar. Look for yourself."

I would not wear a hat to cover the shaved area of my scalp just above my right ear. It only ranged the size of my palm and I wanted to show it off. I was proud of what I had just been through. People would stop and look at me in the grocery store. Of course, I loved this attention and took the opportunity to share my joy in being given this miraculous healing. One of my favorite recantations was of how my surgery had been provided for since most of the public likes to speak poorly about government. I spoke frequently about the generosity of Texas Rehabilitation Commission, and how they had played such a major role in setting me free. Miracles do happen, and it's better to focus on the positive than be in constant complaint about that which does not work accordingly to plan. Of course, one doesn't need a miracle to be positive, but I had plenty to share about.

15. A DIAGNOSIS STANDS

I thought Dr. Willmore was out of his mind with his diagnosis when I visited him one month post-op. I was feeling on top of the world, eager to see my hero. Imagine my shock and dismay when he diagnosed a "textbook case" of clinical depression. "Oh, come off it, Dr. Willmore," I mumbled to myself. He reiterated I had all the signs, straight out of the book: insomnia, euphoria. I couldn't believe him, but my trust for him won out and I took home the prescription he wrote out for an antidepressant. Little did I realize how quickly I would be seeing the full manifestations of major depression in my life.

As I prepared to leave his clinic he smiled at me and stated, "You've been a good patient."

The past tense of that statement was the most impacting as it revealed a closing door. And that door wouldn't be closing if I didn't have full healing. In the midst of my joy I hated to leave him. He had been the whole world to me, had moved mountains for me. Suddenly, it felt like he was patting me on the head like a parent to a toddler with a message saying, "Get on your way." It's a painful experience to have that longstanding relationship severed so quickly. I was just one of many patients to him and he had done his job. Yet, I knew he had affection for me, for my well-being. Now, he had completed his work with me. All that remained were the annual tests for full verification of healing. Suddenly, I had slid down his priority list, and I didn't want to say good-bye.

Tumbling, tumbling…everything around me was falling fast. I was supposed to be in a recuperation phase, but everything was falling fast. I would call Willmore.

"Any seizures?"

"No," I replied.

"You're well then," he reiterated.

And I kept tumbling, tumbling unable to stop the fall.

It was late August, marching into fall. My coping skills had collapsed and so had my marriage. Eric and I were at each other's throats over anything as I had found new skills to stand up and state my mind. I had grown purely reactive as hormones set off, an event Dr. Willmore had not warned me about. Suddenly, I was acting like a teenager, rebellious, and demanding. My breasts were enlarging; my libido had skyrocketed. Adult puberty! Eric didn't know how to handle me, and I was just as surprised as he was. Suddenly, I was gaining a sexual side to myself I had never had access to before. I was overjoyed. The damaged area of my brain had stopped all normal electrical activity in a normal blossoming libido. Now, with my damaged area removed and the electricity flowing with ease I could enjoy the benefits of "normal" for the first time in my life and understand why people became so flushed over sex. This was a new game to me and Eric had a hard time keeping up with me!

By this time, I was beginning to fantasize about hot little red cars. I could hear keys jangling. It's true that I legitimately had to be seizure free for six months in order to pass the state driving test. "Thank God for George Bush," I often exclaimed, or it would be a whole year's wait! By now, my faith in being seizure free had increased to the point that I literally began eyeing hot little red cars though I couldn't conceive of the ability of buying anything on our broken budget. But who knows? Look what the Lord had done for me so far!

Along with my new found adult puberty came rebellion

and defiance, not unlike teenagers. I simply went out of control. I had discovered that I could say 'NO!' instead of my normal sweet compliant act. I was starting to act like Aaron, who was already locked into heavy defiant behaviors. My house became a war zone, Aaron and I locked into deafening clashes, and Eric and Emily withdrawing for sanity.

Following my cravings for red cars, about three or four months post-op, Eric and I began to seek trade-in deals. Eric knew my energy for the wheel would not lend me the patience for learning a stick-shift he already had. So he laid down his own desires at the expense of his wife's cravings. He, too, was eager to see me have my own set of keys to dangle. Within one to two weeks I cast eyes on my dream car and was able to drive it right off the lot, a miracle I just couldn't believe. For weeks, I'd get up at four in the morning and run go look out the window to see if it really was there. Was I really going to be a bona fide driver? Was this a dream? Surely, it couldn't really all be happening.

Once purchase had been made it was Eric's responsibility to teach me major driving skills at age thirty-seven at the only time he had available, evening hours. Thus, we took on the major freeways of Houston. But I was zealous to learn and quick in coordination. This was my burning desire to learn to drive, and this was Eric's courage. For years since, he has regretted telling me to make friends with the accelerator.

As I was practicing driving, I was using my defiance to get my way behind the steering wheel as well as discovering flight on impulse for the first time. I'll never forget the day, a few months into my driver's training, that I discovered the birth of my independence. On that trip I realized I didn't have to give full compliance to his commands to change lanes as he guided me around the Pierce Elevated. I discovered I could use my defiance to get my way behind the steering wheel as well as discovering flight on impulse for the first time. "No," I retorted. "I'll change when I want to change!" I was not dangerous, but I was damned well going to get my way, having been deprived all these years! Of course, this was destructive, but I couldn't see it. I was making up for lost time and counting the days until December 15th, the day I could call myself a legitimate driver. This is when I truly began to lose Eric. How our marriage withstood this time is nothing short of a miracle. But it had to collapse due to the immense dysfunction it was built upon. For me, Eric was only the first of many losses as I saw my life continue to collapse beyond recognition.

By winter, I was broken from isolation. This was supposed to be one of the most joyous times of my life, and in many ways it was, yet I deeply felt as if I was walking in a death. Everything that had been my life was crashing down around me.

I was walking in an immense depression, unable to help myself. I could hardly cope much less function through each day despite this victory of driving. We had no money. There was no place to go. There was no money to spend on entertainment. Formerly dependent on my church for social gathering, I was unable to rejoin weekly activities due to my immense depression. I, of course, did not realize that this was a disorder, and not an emotional dysfunction.

Worsening this and stifling my ability to call out for help was the sexual harassment I received by one of the church members, magnifying the intensity of my sense of victimization. In the aftermath of the encounter I was too fearful to leave my home, and I could certainly not go to the place where I normally encountered this foe, the church! So I closed down completely and begged internally for someone to notice my absence. But no one did. The place where all my contacts were, where I had been married, birthed both children and raised them through preschool, and then poured out my life for over fifteen years seemingly turned its back on me. Months went by and I was not called on. My depression thickened.

Eventually, I did make a call to the church authorities

over the harasser and my inability to overcome my sense of victimization. I begged for support and understanding from the rector, but was received with blank puzzlement. Even my small group leaders shrugged their shoulders at me and quickly changed the topic when I brought up the attack. Since physical rape had not occurred it seemed to them that I was overreacting no matter how psychologically scarring the event had been. One more dependence in my life, the church establishment, had just failed me, and I was fast falling with no one, nothing to stand on. In those days, I sang *On Christ, the Solid Rock I Stand* many times over!

In the midst of that horrible fog of death came December 15th, 1992, six months from my surgical date, the day I could call myself legitimate to drive. I passed the test on the first go round, then had no one to celebrate it with. Eric and I were constantly in heated battle still, and though he was happy for me, our failing relationship dampened what should have been a climactic experience for me. I had never forgotten Dr. Willmore's remarks about throwing me that party when I got my license. When recanting to Eric, he tossed back at me, "If you want something, you have to make it happen." Three days later, after achieving one of my life's dreams, I wrote in my journal, "I don't know who I am anymore. But one thing is sure: All is chaos."

I still had no identity in career. I had been out of the work force for so long that I didn't know who I was at this point. I had exhausted all my unemployment benefits and knew the disgrace of government offices. Somehow, there had to be an answer. I had this marvelous operation offered me. I repeat, I was offered this miraculous healing by Texas Rehabilitation Commission due to the fact that I was so unemployable because of seizures. The seizures are gone. So where am I? Overwhelmed! The creditors were harassing and had been for months. Eric and I were on the verge of losing our house. My explanation story of victorious brain surgery did nothing to those damned creditors. They wanted their money, but I didn't have it. In my overload, my marital collapse, loss of friends, money woes, and joblessness, I cratered and went to a wailing place deep within my soul. I went to my piano.

16. REST AWHILE

It had been standing idle in the corner for twelve or more years. I touched it, played a note. Something happened. The sound beckoned me. A birth of hope.

What could I play? You, my companion. I once knew you so well. But we have been parted so long. How do I draw near to you again?

I didn't know how to approach the keys which I had once hovered so closely over. I had once poured hours a day over this instrument. Now, it was so foreign – yet, so close. I had to pull it close to me. But, I didn't know how.

What music could I play? There was no Bach under my fingers. My fingers were like rust, long forgetting their proper technique. And, furthermore, I didn't care. The pain in my soul only begged to be released.

In my starvation for release, I hauntingly heard Wiley's voice float through my mind over the liquid piano accompaniment of one of the most purifying solo pieces I have ever known. Wiley Beveridge, a college friend, a featured soloist brought light to the dying and hope to the downcast in his presentation of "Rest Awhile" by Stephanie Arje Wood. I must find that score!

The opening a minor arpeggio seemed to pull grief out of me, and I needed no soloist for the piano to display its life. Over the next weeks and months, I couldn't leave that place, the bench. The keys compelled me. The instrument seduced me. I poured out my pain in haunting phrases of mournful passion, grieving as if it wouldn't stop. What had my Lord brought me to? Was not my promise victory? I am broken – broken.

The piece was a monumental discovery to me. It not only brought me back to the piano, but it opened a door of my understanding as to the style of music I was capable of playing. Having been purely classically bred, I could not conceive of playing any alternative style no matter its simplicity. My eyes had just opened and my fingers were absorbing. I was suddenly seeing myself in a role as worship leader, whereas I had always been the follower for years. I instantly saw potential in myself and was amazed at what my future might hold.

Spring '93

17. TRANSFORMATION

As I still battled the torments of depression while suddenly rediscovering my piano, I poured out my torment to a dear sister and church mother, the Rev. Betty Masquelette. She sent me on a silent retreat (God bless her!) at the Villa de Matel not far from my home in response to my torment. This retreat would alter me spiritually in an intense manner, a personal transfiguration of a magnitude only the heart can tell. Never again would I doubt God's personal love for me despite my surrounding issues. The Lord did have a deep word for me on that weekend. At that time, I could hope to see its fruit someday. I can testify to having seen it now! That word was:

"For I know the plans that I have for you," declares the Lord, "plans for welfare and not for calamity to give you a future and a hope.

"Then you will call upon Me and come and pray to Me, and I will listen to you.

"And you will seek Me and find Me, when you search for Me with all your heart.

"And I will be found by you." declares the Lord.

Jer. 29:11-14

It was not until the second day in complete silence that I was able to completely surrender to the Lord. Then, once I had let go, I began to yield my cares and anxieties only to make room for His Spirit of peace and comfort. The Holy Spirit filled me with a depth of love and comfort I had not experienced before although I commonly knew the indwelling of the Holy Spirit. It was during this indwelling, while wandering the grounds of the Villa, that a beautiful transformation began to take place.

The piercing radiance of the presence of the Holy Spirit brought me a nearness to God I had never experienced before. Suddenly, He was all around me. I could see, visually see His Light sparkling in the leaves in the trees, in the dirt beneath my feet where no light had been before. This was no physical light. It was everywhere. And in that Light, I saw that He loved me. I was in His Presence. I saw that He delighted in me, for I was His own. His Presence was all around me like a blanket, covering and protecting me.

Though I walk through the fire – I will not be burned.

I fell back into His arms.

My Father.

I worshipped. I praised. I surrendered again. Then I thanked Him for transforming my eyes, my vision. I knew, at that moment in time and thereafter, His love for me, deep in my heart.

That retreat marked a turning point. It was not, for any stretch of time, the end of my troubles. But the inner strength and grace it gave me to carry over the top are remarkable as compared to the place I was in when entering the Villa. The Lord met me in the lowest place and extended such rich treasure upon me far beyond my knowing. He did not rescue me from the fires I was walking in when I left the Villa that weekend, but I knew, as Paul did in the prison cell, that God loved me, and little else mattered.

Sound simplistic? From the world's standpoint, yes. But the Lord's message to me was plain and simple: focus on His love and I would make it.

The next year things began to turn for me.

"For I know the plans that I have for you, plans for welfare and not for calamity to give you a future and a hope..."
Jer 29:11

POSTLUDE

The fog is lifting. The days are brighter, the nights more rested. The gloom of death has passed, though at times I can still sample its heaviness of yesterday's blackness, its offered defeat. But hope breaks through. I am lighter, able to take on life, ready to seek. The sun is breaking through, profoundly shattering the scope of darkness which has been surrounding me for months. It is time to begin anew.

Part IV

FACING ME

An Identity Waits

It wants to bloom!
It's craving to bloom!

This passion…
Carried internally -
cries out to be heard.

Do I dare to hope?
Can I allow myself to hope?
Can I be heard --
now?

The risk could be too great.
Failure at this level would ruin me.
The performance demands
My innermost expression,
The core of my soul.
It demands my identity.

Can I risk putting my identity on the line?

I have to.

June 1993

18. PLANS FOR ME

The Lord definitely had His plans for me and He began to tell me so right on my own piano! From the time of that silent retreat for the next few months, I was deeply in a spiritual high place and more than ever was compelled to play my piano. This was not Bach and Beethoven, but songs of passion of God's love, expressions of adoration and praise. I had never played piano solo music like this and the therapy in the expression of it, particularly for a trained person such as myself, was easily attainable and rich beyond measure. The music's simplicity drew me back to the core of my love for Him, and pulled out of me my artistry, my passion born in pain.

I could express myself in full artistic means, creating beauty and life at the same time. This therapeutic measure had a number of advantages. It was physically expressive, demanding use of my forearms, wrists, and fingers, an outward release of tension. It was spiritually uplifting in the mere act of praise and thanksgiving, of adoration and love in the midst of trial and bewilderment. And it was free. I could sit endlessly on that bench in free therapy pouring out my pain with automatic release. No psychotherapist could have benefitted me as much, in psyche or my purse, during those months in the spring and summer of 1993. Through this cleansing the Lord began to speak to me. "This is your gift. I have given it to you. I want you to use it."

At this, I would stop playing. "Are You out of Your mind, Lord? It's been twelve years since I've touched this piano! I can't seriously go into this again!"

The music I was playing was an intermediate level, while I had once been well advanced. I now felt Him pulling me to go back to my instrument seriously, but I couldn't conceive of such a notion after such a lengthy time away from my original training. It had been too long. My agility was long gone. And yet, I remembered, Robert Brownlee, my last college piano professor telling me that one never loses it.

"But, Lord," I fought. "That was so long ago. This is not Bach – or Beethoven. You don't know what You're saying!"

I held nothing back from Him.

But I couldn't quench the pull I felt deeply inside. Never before had I felt this way with such a burning desire. I tried to argue Him. Back and forth I explained to Him I had spent seventeen years in accounting and bookkeeping.

The argument thickened. I could not and would not resist playing my piano. It was absolutely addictive to me. The Lord kept pulling me, beckoning me to do more, just what, I didn't know.

"Use it," is all I knew.

That, I could plainly hear.

It was now 1993 and I left music school in 1977. Was He out of His mind? True, I played a little when Aaron was born, but Lord….

Then, one day His truth came to me like lightening. I heard it in the Gospel and from then on, I knew my path was cut. I had to use my gift. My gift was a talent. I had reheard the parable of the talents (Matt 25:14-29), and I was threatened that if I did not use my talent as the Lord had instructed me to He would stifle it. Furthermore, it was clear to me now that it would only increase if I yielded to His instruction though I had no clue in which direction to go. So I yielded to Him. I said, "Yes, Lord; show me where to go. Open the right doors. I know You're behind this. Lead me." And that's just what He began to do.

19. INCREASING TALENTS

How could I doubt the Lord? Even as I pondered on His plans for me, "plans for welfare and not for calamity to give you a future and a hope," Jer. 29:11, the doors were already forming for me to walk through.

It took courage for me to just step out and follow my nose. But that's exactly what I did, not having a clue as to where to start. I can't confess to having any great inspiration of how I was to begin my walk in faith toward using my gift. But after hearing that parable, I knew that I couldn't sit still. I had to act. I began by making a cold call to a local music store, explaining my skills and asked it there was any use for anyone like myself. I carefully explained my strengths of background with full exposure to the time frame I had been away from music. Above all, I believe my enthusiasm for my instrument, my passion for music shone through the detriment of time, and the manager took notice and listened intensely.

My lucky (or blessed) day! It seems the Lord was behind this after all, nudging me the entire way when I couldn't even see it. A woman with a local teaching organization was giving a seminar in two days for interested parties on teaching keyboard skills. Would I be interested?

Teaching keyboard? Isn't this where I started at Sam Houston State all those years ago? This was too good to be true! Now, I have a particular affinity against keyboards versus pianos, but this was the starting place. My students turned out to be a range from toddlers to early elementary children and I found out quickly how much I enjoyed teaching them, for I got as enthused about the music as they did. Even more, I discovered I had a real flare with them. I was amazed to find myself acting in such natural creative skill with them, and my supervisor commented happily at my knack which easily poured out. This completely surprised me within myself, especially with the tensions which were still running so high at home. Yet, with music, I discovered I had real capacity. I could shelve all my worldly concerns, and share the passions of my soul. I wanted these innocent children to fall in love with music just as I had, and it was my job to make it happen. My students got naturally enthused with me, and we all had fun together cheering each other on. Everybody had a good time. It was a wonderful setting in which to lay a foundation.

There was only one factor in my new career which was unsatisfactory. I drove from school to school to teach in the after-school programs, a different school each day. But, as I began to take on elementary age children and see them flourish under my direction solely in group settings, my appetite could not be quenched with simple group direction. I wanted to be a private teacher and I wanted it passionately. I loved working with these children and they responded to me well. Could I possibly be a private teacher? How did one go about becoming one, knowing the repertoire for the various levels? With my huge memory gaps from my epileptic years, I could hardly remember any of my primary or intermediate teaching. My memory started with the Anna Magdalena Notebook of Johann Sebastian Bach, well into intermediate instruction. As teachers of practical methods know, we teach so much by our experience; we simply pass on the heritage of what we have been given. How could I pass on my heritage when my memory had failed me previously? I needed to find the stepping stones, but was embarrassed at my situation. I needed to find out how to be a teacher. I had no confidence in my abilities intact other than what I had seen at a very primary level, which was that my character was a very good match. Somehow, I needed to find help.

My teaching ability in music was not the only talent the Lord was revealing to me at this time. He was also improving my performance skills for I had taken a position as Music Director at a local church near our home. I suppose that once I had let surgeons drill holes in my skull and enter my brain, I got a little bold. Never had I performed before, but I was stepping out and gaining new confidence. Suddenly, I was believing in myself and acting in like method by selling myself to others. This would not have happened two years ago!

Making it clear I was no organist, the selection team was most happy with my Bach and hired me instantly despite my lack of choral experience. I explained I had many years, more than I could count, within choirs, but not directing. However, my music school background swayed them. I also noticed I was beginning to sound more confident and persuasive as I talked. This was a new blossoming confidence which utterly surprised me!

Learning to play in front of a congregation after years of silence was a major coming out. Even in my preliminary days I would only let Eric listen to me as a freshman through the time I left the music school. So taking this step was awesome, preparing new work every week, suddenly calling up every skill I had ever been trained for. My world was suddenly surrounded by music and I felt happy by it. My piano technique was expanding, old skills were returning. Then one day, while goofing around on the organ, I suddenly realized I was playing a piece by memory I had not played since I was sixteen.

My fingers delightfully poured out J. S. Bach's Invention XIV in full detail, not missing a note. The score was at home in my library. I had glanced at it once earlier on the piano at home, then stuffed the score back in my music library. Prior that playing, I was sixteen when I last was familiar with the notes.

That was the day I knew my memory had gone through major recovery, retaining data it never could have recalled pre-op. I called Dr. Willmore's office enthusiastically to report my happy news as soon as I got home.

Fall-Winter 1993

20. FACING ME

When I found Betty in the fall of '94, she forced me to look in the mirror of reality, which meant ability, potential, and strength. She would not stand for me to use such characteristics of bondage, inability, and victimization in my overtones of explanation of myself. Although I had gained momentum in finding a sense of capacity, a tangible start to a possible career, it was but a mere foothold. I embarrassingly tried to explain to her my list of deficits in memory defects. She would cut me off immediately with, "What makes you think you can't...?" She did all this on my first visit with her. Betty J. Shaw, Director of Piano Pedagogy at the University of Houston's Moores School of Music was referred to me by someone knowing I wanted to know more about teaching. I went to her in fear and trembling (she will laugh to remember), begging to audit a course. What did I know about teaching, other than I wanted to? Upon explaining my story to this kind, motherly woman who genuinely seemed warm and tender, she told me that a family member of hers had epilepsy. She had seen seizures. Then she truly did understand! She didn't cower away from me as so much of the general public had, or look at me with strange quizzical eyes. Instead, she seemed to embrace me in her heart. I immediately felt attachment to her. She didn't seem afraid to speak of it the way most of the general public is, even if it was history to me. It had been so much of me for so long, my past memory difficulty still, that it was still very important. Betty gave me permission for the course and I grew very excited.

Through Betty, I took on my first private students. Every question, every doubt went straight to my mentor and she spent months filing away at my attitude, adjusting the "can't" spirit insisting that, "Yes, you can!" I began to see for myself that she was right. I had no right to be so hard on myself. I began to stand on my own confidence for the first time. In this manner, Betty Shaw was every bit just as much a hero to me as Dr. Willmore was. Dr. Willmore healed me physically but left me psychologically in a slump unable to rise and start my life again. As indebted as I am to this dear man, it is imperative to realize the fullness of the psychological identity that consumes the epileptic. Without the sense of being able to rise again over one's own negative mindset of defeat one is still locked in a box even without seizures. By God's grace and leading, I met Betty, and she opened my box.

A woman of more compassion and more patience than I will ever understand, Betty endured my strongest arguments, then gently led me back to the truth, "Yes, you are good enough, and better than that." Why did I doubt myself so much? Of course, her love was so addicting I couldn't resist. This sort of belief in me was so attractive I couldn't turn away. How could she claim to know me so well? Over and over, I wanted to doubt her. I had only walked into her life a few months ago. Why was she giving so much of her time to me? Who was I to her? But she continued to call me at night to check on me, to encourage me with my students, and to talk to me of personal issues. She was fast becoming like a mother to me, the close, personal, warm relationship I had always wanted but never had with my own mother. And so my heart beat the day at her kitchen table where we so often met when she placed her hand on mine and told me I was her adopted daughter. From then on, I have claimed her as my adopted mother, for she is far more than mentor to me. Betty simply took up where my doctor had left off until I could stand up completely on my own. For her, I am just as deeply indebted as to Dr. Willmore.

21. PERFECT POSTER PERSON

A monumental event was on the horizon that would cast out any remains of my self-doubt that Betty Shaw hadn't already been able to reach. Through her, my personal relationships were healing, including my marriage. My self-awareness had come intact and was in formation stages; and I was in the enjoyment stages with a career for the first time of my life. I had left the church position over political overtures and was now solely devoted to my students. These were growing regularly under Betty's direction and her new leads. I taught at her home in a back studio, and I loved having access to Betty in between students. She taught and I taught, then we often conferred later that evening. It was a wonderful environment to nurture my skill, and I truly saw my students flourish.

I saw my ability to be creative with them spontaneously. This was not a taught skill. It was a teacher's gift. But most of all, I saw the gift of encouragement. Never having received this as a child, I was awed when I found myself using praise and encouragement with my students. Betty's 'win' spirit was wearing off on me, my passion for music was prevailing, and I wanted these young tender students to fall in love with music just as I had. Nothing must dampen their spirit.

Under Betty's guidance, I had made contact with Robert Brownlee, my former piano professor, who was still on staff at the University of Houston. For her to get me to do this, she literally had to march me down to the main academic building at the university. Of course, I had no tuition monies, nor faith despite the sequence of events which were already taking place. Through Betty's hand-holding, I secured a small student loan for a year's part-time load, and began full piano studies again. Even so, I had the same professor that I had twenty years previously, just as brilliant as ever, with the same magnificent Bösendorfer piano I had fallen in love with years ago. It was all coming to pass and my talent would be developed just as the Lord had instructed me.

It was three years after my surgery and I received a phone call one day from the neuropsychological department at the UT Med School stating they wanted a reassessment as a follow-up to my brain surgery. No cost.

I had seen remarkable memory improvement in those past years and noticed a keen curiosity in things around me. Despite the odds Eric and I were still trying to sort out in our marriage, I was high in perseverance, constantly collecting new "old data" from sudden new memory hitting me, and I was on a search for myself. Something monumental was happening to my life; I could feel it. I had a vividness about me that had never been before, and a great sense of a great awakening. It was difficult to explain to Eric. For months, it just seemed that something monumental was in the midst of occurring . I could feel it. Perhaps it was rewiring. I just knew something BIG was happening. So when I got that phone call I knew I would have a chance to find out what had happened to my brain overall since the right temporal lobectomy.

Before the results came in the doctors were amazed when I completed their six-hour battery of tests in two hours, and they told me so. They seemed ecstatic, yet it would be another week before I knew anything concrete in their results. They assured me they would call me right away, and that I would be very pleased.

"You are the perfect Poster-Person. What we all hope for." Dr. Joshua Breier, Ph.D. Clinical Neuropsychologist had just read my test results to me. My Full Scale, Verbal, and Performance IQ's had leapt up by 24 points each, verifying what I had been experiencing in my day to day routine. Dr.

Breier continued to assess that I was now at the high end of the superior range in full scale IQ near Mensa quality. This was more than I could fathom. The news was too great to contain. Suddenly, I found myself blurting out from out of the blue, "I want to go back to school!"

I had not thought of school in years. Piano, yes. Refining my teaching skills, to be certain. But school? A degree?

"Why don't you?" quickly encouraged Dr. Breier. "You could go anywhere you want to go. You could do anything you want to do!"

But I have no money, I thought. And defeat wanted to catch me in its trap.

As I departed the hospital, thanking the doctor, I wondered where my comment had come from. I had not thought of school in years! Where did this silly notion come from? But never mind. I was elated I had lost nothing when they took out the right temporal lobe. So I walked to my hot little red car parked in Hermann Park, thankful beyond measure and still baffled at my comment over school. All I could do was release this to the Lord. "Lord, if You want me to go back to school *You* do it! You open the doors. You know I have no money. You know I have no way to make this happen, but if You want it, You do it!" And with that, I released it, falling into ecstatic praise for my wonderful results. Meanwhile, a blessing was already unfolding.

22. PLANS FOR WELFARE

Three days later, JoAnn Hoffmann, former president of the Houston Music Teachers Association, walked up to me at the Memorial Piano Teachers Association annual spring luncheon and asked me, "Aren't you that student under Betty Shaw attending the University of Houston?"

I responded, "I've audited a class under Betty, but I'm not a student there."

JoAnn then extended, "I know of some scholarship funds available. Would you be interested?"

It was as simple as that, and it's a miracle I didn't faint on the spot.

"I know the plans that I have for you, plans for welfare, and not for calamity..." Jer. 29:11

My first course of action was disbelief, but JoAnn, with her genuine enthusiasm and encouragement, went on to prove the meaning behind her words. She was the force behind the Education Foundation within HMTA. So far, no one had used the funds. She would be glad to have a recipient.

Me? Going back to school? At mid-life? Betty jumped in instantly and assured me the campus was full of older students. Eric was excited as well. I admit to being a bit frightened of that sprawling campus, but with such high IQ scores, I felt I could prove anything, tackle the world. After all, Dr. Breier had said I could do anything!

23. TESTING MY LIMITS

I didn't count on having to take algebra or geology or two years of foreign language when I went back to music school. If I had not gained a winning spirit, a belief in my ability to overcome obstacles, my path would have stopped dead end. But my sense of endurance outlived confusion, and I was pleased to find myself continually on the Dean's List, an academic rating I had never known in my previous schooling.

I enjoyed classes at this stage of my life. History and English essays took on complete new life that I never appreciated at age twenty. I was fascinated for the most part with my subject studies (except geology). I wanted to see how far my brain could take me. I had never enjoyed college this way directly out of high school. I am certain some of my maturity added to my improved attitude, but I never lost the constant running tape in the back of my mind of the doctors telling me of my superior improvement. Yet, more than a tape, my alertness had drastically improved, and I was really enjoying this. My one gripe about school was the constant roll of friction in younger students who griped about having to do this assignment or that assignment. They seemed to be missing the point for which we were all gathered.

I was enjoying the research and the expansion mode. The discovery of new elements of truth was meaningful to me, even if it was outside my immediate field. I was particularly moved by reading a book about a Native American for an English assignment, and suddenly relating to the great injustice done to this mighty people. Never had I seen this in such a light. I could easily relate the two injustices, whether they be race or health disorder in my case. We must guard against supremacy, I thought, or we fracture ourselves into broken pieces with no strength.

My studio grew rapidly as my confidence soared and my pleasure in teaching mounted. My motherhood experiences paid off with my students; but mostly it was Betty's winning spirit that gave me success. Giving my students that spirit of "Yes, you can," is my greatest joy, and is a direct product of Betty Shaw. No students hitting themselves on the head for the sake of stupidity in my studio!

Two years into my piano and course studies, my scholarship with Houston Music Teachers Association, Education Foundation expired. I still had about two years course work left since the first years had only been part-time. Once again, I went to Betty, who I was seeing weekly in her home and studio as I taught. She had an idea. Of course! I knew I could count on Betty.

Betty wanted me to audition for a scholarship directly with the Moores School of Music at the University of Houston. "Now, Betty," I revolted, "that's just for the top performers. I can play the piano, but I'm no performer." Still, she insisted. So, I faithfully set a date for an audition, shaking in my shoes, wondering what I was doing, and trusting there had to be some rhyme and reason to it. I had begun work on several selections which would end up in my recital, and I chose those to play.

My audition was on a Saturday. Friday, I received the word.

My beloved paternal grandmother, Lil, the one family member who had always nurtured me on the piano, had just died. Lil and I had been very bonded, especially in my early years at Sam Houston State. My most cherished memory of her was her delight in hearing me play when my own family of origin took no interest at all. In those days at Sam, when my weekends were spent with her, she'd seat herself on her couch near the piano and simply ask me to play. Now, that cherished memory was going to sail me through my scholarship audition.

I was shaky walking onto the stage the next day to meet the grand Steinway. News of Lil's death had taken its toll on me. Betty had assured me she would inform the staff, but I knew I was not on top of myself. Inside, I wanted to collapse.

In the back row of Dudley recital hall sat all of the members of the piano faculty waiting to hear my melodious sounds. This was my one chance. Emotions could not get in my way. So I sat down on that bench, prayed inside my soul, pictured Lil, and played for her. The music was beautiful as I gave way to her. I played with all my soul for Lil, who was sitting there like a lady, as she was, lapping in the beauty. All the faculty was lost to me. The stage was lost to me. I had only one thing to do. Play for Lil.

Within a few weeks came the official letter from the Moores School. I had won the scholarship.

The scholarship turned me into a full time student, twelve course hours per semester. By now, I was also carrying twenty-five students per week. This on top of preparing for my senior recital, but I was loving it! I had won the scholarship, the students loved me, and I loved them. Isn't this the life that was intended for me all along?

I was fast closing in on completing all my course work and knowing I was at the point of reaching my ultimate goal, the recital. This was the last step in order to complete my degree plan. I would then have achieved that which I set out to do so long ago. Mr. Brownlee and I had chosen a program, a challenging one. I was in the midst of preparation. Could my dream really be that close? Could I really reach this mountaintop?

24. THE UNTHINKABLE

Spring 1997. The priest standing at the front of the room where the education meeting is being held is sounding louder and louder. Seated around a large conference table I want him to shut up! I can't understand my reaction. Randall is a remarkably peaceful presenter, filled with empathy as he explains the subject matter over human relationships. Despite his softness, his voice seems to be penetrating a wall within that is on the verge of crumbling. My resistance to his voice has suddenly grown remarkably thin and I do not understand why. Stop! Please, stop! But, I dare not, nor can I call out his name. I do not understand why I am feeling this way. He is only explaining the regular criteria for the meeting. My feeling of resistance toward sound grows, "Stop, Randall, stop!"

Minutes later, a time span I do not know, I hear my name called out, "Stephanie, can you hear me?"

I am on the floor under the table.

I am dazed, disoriented.

I am told I have had a seizure.

Someone is going after Eric.

Annie is at my side. Annie is a nurse. As I gain consciousness, I emotionally revolt. *No! I scream. I cannot have a seizure!* But, I am still disoriented, in a deep fog. Only in the deep recesses of my mind did I actually scream. Yet, that is where I live my nightmare. I am wild with fury, panicked out of my still dazed mind. I cannot be sedated. I will not be comforted. The other meeting participants have been led away. I cannot think. I cannot see, only relive the horror of isolation and rejection as, once again, I am secluded from everyone who claims to be loving. As Randall put it to me months later, "What could they do?"

The discomfort of watching another person go through

a rigorous convulsion was far greater for the crowd watching than for the one having the seizure or convulsion, I later found out. It was easier to file out of the room and carry on in a different place than to meet the problem head on in courage with understanding and sympathy. I soared back to my early childhood memories of being "removed promptly and isolated until I returned to sanity."(p.14) Since I could not be removed due to the limpness of my leg and torso, the group simply filed out, leaving me grappling in rejection as a discard. Annie, of course, stayed. There was one other assistant from the group. But I wanted to feel my brothers' and sisters' arms around me, accepting and encouraging me for being a part of their ministry. The isolation meant rejection to me. I panicked. No! No! Only Eric's arrival could bring me to any kind of resting-place.

Eric always knew how to handle me regarding seizures. He embraced and caressed me as I wanted the whole world to do. I could not walk, my left side completely limp. Finally, he semi-carried me out of the building. I believe there was a wheelchair used. Then he took me home and put me to bed. We could do nothing until morning when we could call Dr. Willmore's office.

Damn it! Don't you know he was out of town again! Willmore has this uncanny way of being out of town when I need him the most. I made an immediate appointment with an understudy of Dr. Willmore's and proceeded to have a MRI as well. The testing was clean, but the office visit unsatisfactory. I could give no account of the seizure, of the intensity of its load, due to my unconsciousness, and when the intern heard my lack of symptoms, she decided I had a panic attack. I fought her diagnosis but could give no description of my actual behavior due to my unconsciousness. She kept blankly staring at me, then dismissed me for my lack of verbal description. Panic attack it was, no matter what I said, and this was her report to Dr. Willmore. It was not until months later, many seizures later, and a written account from Annie that Dr. Willmore finally believed I had started to have some form of seizure activity appear. For months, he tossed it off as panic attacks due to that first wretched office visit and an intern who didn't have listening skills. Then, of course, Dr. Willmore wanted to believe that I had been healed completely. After all, it had been five years without medicine. What happened?

Suddenly, every eight weeks, there they were, but different, not in the form of a staring spell. This time the seizures were generalized, grabbing my entire body but not my consciousness. So I watched in horror as my body thrashed, hearing myself grunting like a monkey. Mentally, I anguished over the lack of response my body was giving me though I was determined to control it. I could not. I'd feel myself wanting to cry from despair, but my glands couldn't pass a tear, were somehow inoperable. The worst part, I believe, is never knowing when the chaos would end or *if* it would end. I have often described it to friends as like opening an airplane hatch mid-air and finding yourself falling, falling, falling…not knowing….

"What should I do?" someone asked.

I responded, "Take my hand. Assure me that you are there. Don't leave me. I don't know when I'm coming down. Please don't leave me. Turn me on my side. Bring me water afterward. Let me know by your presence that I'm going to have a safe landing."

The one fortunate characteristic of this new type of seizure which was eventually found to be controllable through medication was its strong aura. I was given several minutes warning when it did decide to hit. I was fortunate to have this "window shade" warning for the sake of safety. The "window shade" warning was a simple change in my cognizance for a split second. It was as if the blinds were suddenly being drawn tightly shut, then opened bright again. At this point, I knew I had better run for cover, grab some Adivan, solicit help, and lay down in the nearest place possible. Usually I had three minutes or so before the convulsing would actually start. What others don't realize in many generalized seizures such as I was having is that I could hear everything around me. I was aware of my surroundings to a degree, but was totally unable to communicate nor command my body. I did not always lose consciousness depending on the medicine strength I was on. For this reason, I have always asked that my family members reassure me and talk to me kindly while I am in such a traumatic experience. It is truly like being in hell itself.

It was finally proven through an EEG that some leftover scar tissue near the hypothalamus area from the lobectomy was triggering the activity. Today, after several years of adjustments with medications and fighting stifling side-effects, the seizures are controlled. They are certainly no longer a threat and I live fully with no regard to thought to their interruption.

25. BELIEVE IN YOURSELF

Believe in yourself, and in your plan,
Say not, "I cannot," but say "I can."
Most prizes of life we fail to win,
Because we doubt the power within.

AUTHOR UNKNOWN

Believe in yourself. How could I continue to believe in myself with this ghost from my past threatening to disqualify me? The ghost ranted out, "Not good enough…poor memory…undependable." Didn't I know this voice well? How easy it was to follow! The defeat I felt at the reoccurrence of these rare seizure episodes threatened my complete image which the Lord had been turning around for the past years.

No! I couldn't let it happen! I had been brought too far! It was all in the mindset and I had to make a decision. I had to keep on believing, to stand in my faith and in what my Father had already shown me. "I have a plan for you...plans for welfare…."

I had already seen the beginning of the outcome of this plan. I must persist.

I now knew that those seizures would not defeat me, would not define me. I came to this conclusion fortunately before the seizures were controlled, when they were occurring about every eight weeks. Now, I give thanksgiving for the control, but my restoration came in knowing God's calling on me which is a multiple purpose.

I knew that I was to keep going in music. I knew that I was to keep teaching. I must not let this blow deter me from the recital, which lay immediately in from of me, and of which I had dreamed for so long.

Going back on medication one year in front of my senior recital was a severe blow. Would I allow the set-back that my memory would now suffer from drugs to throw me back into a mode of defeat? I had overcome so much, gained such great distances, and yet I immediately felt ambushed by those drugs and their affects on my memory. How could I pull this recital off as a serious artist? I knew in my own history what the meds would do to me.

My creativity won the battle once more as I pondered the obstacle in front of me. I believe it was Betty's, "Yes, you can," which had been internalized by now, that was taking me by the hand. To play at Dudley Recital Hall would certainly mean full memorized scores. I struggled mightily with this, even considering doctor's excuses which Mr. Brownlee flatly turned down. Then I thought of Clarence.

One of my more advanced adult students, a CEO, Clarence Comer, had just bought a concert Steinway grand the year before for his back parlor. *I'll give my recital there.* I thought. *As his teacher, he'll be glad to accommodate me.* In this way I could use the scores, have a more intimate recital, and be thrilled with the piano. Clarence was most happy to yield his home to me for the occasion. The recital, my grand coming-out, finally occurred in May 1998. It was a mountaintop experience for me, a summit which had been blocked for most of my life. When it was as all over after a year and a half of working up to this point, I thought, *I wish I could do it all over again.* This dream had become a reality, and only by believing in myself with hard dedication and grueling application had I been able to make it happen.

One year later in 1999, I graduated from the Moores School of Music, another unfolding dream turned reality. This happened mid-life for me at age 44 when most of my age set was in the bleachers watching their children march to "Pomp and Circumstance." It didn't matter to me. I had finally attained my goal. My mission, just as the plaque on my piano says, is to pass onto my students that belief in one's self. We are bigger than our obstacles, or the Lord will show us how to deal with them. We must reach deep within because He will always meet us there. Hope is ours is we will take it and believe. Now it is mine to give back what has so wonderfully been given to me.

CONCLUSION

I was given the immense gift of God's love personified through three wonderful people. Only in this way could the stream of negativity and rejection be broken that had been a constant source of intake from my youth. Only in this way could I begin to see God's love for myself in such magnitude that hope was born, and can now be returned to others. Those three, Eric, Dr. Willmore, and Betty Shaw, I am eternally grateful for. Those three have been beams of a greater mission. The first, Eric, was my discovered safe place. The second, Dr. Willmore, was the power to reach for a star, and the third, Betty, was the power to break old habits of disbelief. Yes, Betty, I can!

As this power has come to me, I now pass it on. It is my thrill in daily events to pass it to my piano students who walk in my door with looks of dismay crying out, "Mrs. Sawyer, this is too hard!" But when they leave, they are enlightened by their own ability, not by what I have done, but in what they have discovered for themselves.

Sadly, the foes of ignorance in dealing with seizures are still highly active in the public at large. I still run into discrimination as a public servant with my music skills. If someone hears of a seizure, even if remote, they become afraid and don't want me around. People still want to accuse in false terms such as possession of spirit. It has happened to me countless times. I believe that only in educating the general public will we be able to break these strongholds. It is only in bonding together in love and acceptance that we make ourselves a better society, not by casting out in rejection through fear. One woman cried out to me, "Not in front of the children!" thereby releasing her fear of a possible invasion. If we teach our children bias we are not teaching them love. And if we are afraid, we are not believing in our own abilities to love and accept, to show the way.

Printed in the United States
5856